I Am
What I Eat

This Is What I Ate

Inspire Publishing

Date: ___________________________

Breakfast

	Calories	Carbs	Protein	Fats
_______________________				
_______________________				
_______________________				
_______________________				

Lunch

	Calories	Carbs	Protein	Fats
_______________________				
_______________________				
_______________________				
_______________________				

Snacks

	Calories	Carbs	Protein	Fats
_______________________				
_______________________				
_______________________				
_______________________				

Dinner

	Calories	Carbs	Protein	Fats
_______________________				
_______________________				
_______________________				
_______________________				

	Calories	Carbs	Protein	Fats
Totals				

Cups of Water Today

Date: _______________________

Breakfast

	Calories	Carbs	Protein	Fats
_________________________				
_________________________				
_________________________				
_________________________				

Lunch

	Calories	Carbs	Protein	Fats
_________________________				
_________________________				
_________________________				
_________________________				

Snacks

	Calories	Carbs	Protein	Fats
_________________________				
_________________________				
_________________________				
_________________________				

Dinner

	Calories	Carbs	Protein	Fats
_________________________				
_________________________				
_________________________				
_________________________				

	Calories	Carbs	Protein	Fats
Totals				

Cups of Water Today

Date: _______________________

Breakfast

		Calories	Carbs	Protein	Fats
________________		☐	☐	☐	☐
________________		☐	☐	☐	☐
________________		☐	☐	☐	☐
________________		☐	☐	☐	☐

Lunch

		Calories	Carbs	Protein	Fats
________________		☐	☐	☐	☐
________________		☐	☐	☐	☐
________________		☐	☐	☐	☐
________________		☐	☐	☐	☐

Snacks

		Calories	Carbs	Protein	Fats
________________		☐	☐	☐	☐
________________		☐	☐	☐	☐
________________		☐	☐	☐	☐
________________		☐	☐	☐	☐

Dinner

		Calories	Carbs	Protein	Fats
________________		☐	☐	☐	☐
________________		☐	☐	☐	☐
________________		☐	☐	☐	☐
________________		☐	☐	☐	☐

	Calories	Carbs	Protein	Fats
Totals	☐	☐	☐	☐

Cups of Water Today

Date: ______________________

Breakfast

	Calories	Carbs	Protein	Fats
____________________				
____________________				
____________________				
____________________				

Lunch

	Calories	Carbs	Protein	Fats
____________________				
____________________				
____________________				
____________________				

Snacks

	Calories	Carbs	Protein	Fats
____________________				
____________________				
____________________				
____________________				

Dinner

	Calories	Carbs	Protein	Fats
____________________				
____________________				
____________________				
____________________				

	Calories	Carbs	Protein	Fats
Totals				

Cups of Water Today

Date: ________________________

Breakfast

	Calories	Carbs	Protein	Fats
__________________________				
__________________________				
__________________________				
__________________________				

Lunch

	Calories	Carbs	Protein	Fats
__________________________				
__________________________				
__________________________				
__________________________				

Snacks

	Calories	Carbs	Protein	Fats
__________________________				
__________________________				
__________________________				
__________________________				

Dinner

	Calories	Carbs	Protein	Fats
__________________________				
__________________________				
__________________________				
__________________________				

	Calories	Carbs	Protein	Fats
Totals				

Cups of Water Today

Date: _______________________

Breakfast

	Calories	Carbs	Protein	Fats
______________________				
______________________				
______________________				
______________________				

Lunch

	Calories	Carbs	Protein	Fats
______________________				
______________________				
______________________				
______________________				

Snacks

	Calories	Carbs	Protein	Fats
______________________				
______________________				
______________________				
______________________				

Dinner

	Calories	Carbs	Protein	Fats
______________________				
______________________				
______________________				
______________________				

	Calories	Carbs	Protein	Fats
Totals				

Cups of Water Today

Date: _______________________

Breakfast

	Calories	Carbs	Protein	Fats
____________________				
____________________				
____________________				
____________________				

Lunch

	Calories	Carbs	Protein	Fats
____________________				
____________________				
____________________				
____________________				

Snacks

	Calories	Carbs	Protein	Fats
____________________				
____________________				
____________________				
____________________				

Dinner

	Calories	Carbs	Protein	Fats
____________________				
____________________				
____________________				
____________________				

	Calories	Carbs	Protein	Fats
Totals				

Cups of Water Today

Date: _______________________

Breakfast

	Calories	Carbs	Protein	Fats
_________________________				
_________________________				
_________________________				
_________________________				

Lunch

	Calories	Carbs	Protein	Fats
_________________________				
_________________________				
_________________________				
_________________________				

Snacks

	Calories	Carbs	Protein	Fats
_________________________				
_________________________				
_________________________				
_________________________				

Dinner

	Calories	Carbs	Protein	Fats
_________________________				
_________________________				
_________________________				
_________________________				

	Calories	Carbs	Protein	Fats
Totals				

Cups of Water Today

Date: _______________________

Breakfast

	Calories	Carbs	Protein	Fats
___________________________				
___________________________				
___________________________				
___________________________				

Lunch

	Calories	Carbs	Protein	Fats
___________________________				
___________________________				
___________________________				
___________________________				

Snacks

	Calories	Carbs	Protein	Fats
___________________________				
___________________________				
___________________________				
___________________________				

Dinner

	Calories	Carbs	Protein	Fats
___________________________				
___________________________				
___________________________				
___________________________				

	Calories	Carbs	Protein	Fats
Totals				

Cups of Water Today

Date: ___________________________

Breakfast

	Calories	Carbs	Protein	Fats
_______________________				
_______________________				
_______________________				
_______________________				

Lunch

	Calories	Carbs	Protein	Fats
_______________________				
_______________________				
_______________________				
_______________________				

Snacks

	Calories	Carbs	Protein	Fats
_______________________				
_______________________				
_______________________				
_______________________				

Dinner

	Calories	Carbs	Protein	Fats
_______________________				
_______________________				
_______________________				
_______________________				

	Calories	Carbs	Protein	Fats
Totals				

Cups of Water Today

Date: _______________________

Breakfast

	Calories	Carbs	Protein	Fats
_________________________				
_________________________				
_________________________				
_________________________				

Lunch

	Calories	Carbs	Protein	Fats
_________________________				
_________________________				
_________________________				
_________________________				

Snacks

	Calories	Carbs	Protein	Fats
_________________________				
_________________________				
_________________________				
_________________________				

Dinner

	Calories	Carbs	Protein	Fats
_________________________				
_________________________				
_________________________				
_________________________				

	Calories	Carbs	Protein	Fats
Totals				

Cups of Water Today

Date: ___________________________

Breakfast

	Calories	Carbs	Protein	Fats
_____________________				
_____________________				
_____________________				
_____________________				

Lunch

	Calories	Carbs	Protein	Fats
_____________________				
_____________________				
_____________________				
_____________________				

Snacks

	Calories	Carbs	Protein	Fats
_____________________				
_____________________				
_____________________				
_____________________				

Dinner

	Calories	Carbs	Protein	Fats
_____________________				
_____________________				
_____________________				
_____________________				

	Calories	Carbs	Protein	Fats
Totals				

Cups of Water Today

Date: _________________________

Breakfast

	Calories	Carbs	Protein	Fats
________________________				
________________________				
________________________				
________________________				

Lunch

	Calories	Carbs	Protein	Fats
________________________				
________________________				
________________________				
________________________				

Snacks

	Calories	Carbs	Protein	Fats
________________________				
________________________				
________________________				
________________________				

Dinner

	Calories	Carbs	Protein	Fats
________________________				
________________________				
________________________				
________________________				

	Calories	Carbs	Protein	Fats
Totals				

Cups of Water Today

Date: _______________________

Breakfast

	Calories	Carbs	Protein	Fats
____________________________				
____________________________				
____________________________				
____________________________				

Lunch

	Calories	Carbs	Protein	Fats
____________________________				
____________________________				
____________________________				
____________________________				

Snacks

	Calories	Carbs	Protein	Fats
____________________________				
____________________________				
____________________________				
____________________________				

Dinner

	Calories	Carbs	Protein	Fats
____________________________				
____________________________				
____________________________				
____________________________				

	Calories	Carbs	Protein	Fats
Totals				

Cups of Water Today

Date: ______________________

Breakfast

	Calories	Carbs	Protein	Fats
______________________				
______________________				
______________________				
______________________				

Lunch

	Calories	Carbs	Protein	Fats
______________________				
______________________				
______________________				
______________________				

Snacks

	Calories	Carbs	Protein	Fats
______________________				
______________________				
______________________				
______________________				

Dinner

	Calories	Carbs	Protein	Fats
______________________				
______________________				
______________________				
______________________				

	Calories	Carbs	Protein	Fats
Totals				

Cups of Water Today

Date: ___________________

Breakfast

	Calories	Carbs	Protein	Fats
________________________	☐	☐	☐	☐
________________________	☐	☐	☐	☐
________________________	☐	☐	☐	☐
________________________	☐	☐	☐	☐

Lunch

	Calories	Carbs	Protein	Fats
________________________	☐	☐	☐	☐
________________________	☐	☐	☐	☐
________________________	☐	☐	☐	☐
________________________	☐	☐	☐	☐

Snacks

	Calories	Carbs	Protein	Fats
________________________	☐	☐	☐	☐
________________________	☐	☐	☐	☐
________________________	☐	☐	☐	☐
________________________	☐	☐	☐	☐

Dinner

	Calories	Carbs	Protein	Fats
________________________	☐	☐	☐	☐
________________________	☐	☐	☐	☐
________________________	☐	☐	☐	☐
________________________	☐	☐	☐	☐

	Calories	Carbs	Protein	Fats
Totals	☐	☐	☐	☐

Cups of Water Today

Date: _______________________

Breakfast

	Calories	Carbs	Protein	Fats
____________________				
____________________				
____________________				
____________________				

Lunch

	Calories	Carbs	Protein	Fats
____________________				
____________________				
____________________				
____________________				

Snacks

	Calories	Carbs	Protein	Fats
____________________				
____________________				
____________________				
____________________				

Dinner

	Calories	Carbs	Protein	Fats
____________________				
____________________				
____________________				
____________________				

	Calories	Carbs	Protein	Fats
Totals				

Cups of Water Today

Date: _______________________

Breakfast

	Calories	Carbs	Protein	Fats
_______________________	☐	☐	☐	☐
_______________________	☐	☐	☐	☐
_______________________	☐	☐	☐	☐
_______________________	☐	☐	☐	☐

Lunch

	Calories	Carbs	Protein	Fats
_______________________	☐	☐	☐	☐
_______________________	☐	☐	☐	☐
_______________________	☐	☐	☐	☐
_______________________	☐	☐	☐	☐

Snacks

	Calories	Carbs	Protein	Fats
_______________________	☐	☐	☐	☐
_______________________	☐	☐	☐	☐
_______________________	☐	☐	☐	☐
_______________________	☐	☐	☐	☐

Dinner

	Calories	Carbs	Protein	Fats
_______________________	☐	☐	☐	☐
_______________________	☐	☐	☐	☐
_______________________	☐	☐	☐	☐
_______________________	☐	☐	☐	☐

	Calories	Carbs	Protein	Fats
Totals	☐	☐	☐	☐

Cups of Water Today

Date: _______________________

Breakfast

	Calories	Carbs	Protein	Fats
_______________________				
_______________________				
_______________________				
_______________________				

Lunch

	Calories	Carbs	Protein	Fats
_______________________				
_______________________				
_______________________				
_______________________				

Snacks

	Calories	Carbs	Protein	Fats
_______________________				
_______________________				
_______________________				
_______________________				

Dinner

	Calories	Carbs	Protein	Fats
_______________________				
_______________________				
_______________________				
_______________________				

	Calories	Carbs	Protein	Fats
Totals				

Cups of Water Today

Date: ______________________

Breakfast

	Calories	Carbs	Protein	Fats
_______________________				
_______________________				
_______________________				
_______________________				

Lunch

	Calories	Carbs	Protein	Fats
_______________________				
_______________________				
_______________________				
_______________________				

Snacks

	Calories	Carbs	Protein	Fats
_______________________				
_______________________				
_______________________				
_______________________				

Dinner

	Calories	Carbs	Protein	Fats
_______________________				
_______________________				
_______________________				
_______________________				

	Calories	Carbs	Protein	Fats
Totals				

Cups of Water Today

Date: ___________________________

Breakfast

	Calories	Carbs	Protein	Fats
________________________				
________________________				
________________________				
________________________				

Lunch

	Calories	Carbs	Protein	Fats
________________________				
________________________				
________________________				
________________________				

Snacks

	Calories	Carbs	Protein	Fats
________________________				
________________________				
________________________				
________________________				

Dinner

	Calories	Carbs	Protein	Fats
________________________				
________________________				
________________________				
________________________				

	Calories	Carbs	Protein	Fats
Totals				

Cups of Water Today

Date: _________________________

Breakfast

	Calories	Carbs	Protein	Fats
_________________________				
_________________________				
_________________________				
_________________________				

Lunch

	Calories	Carbs	Protein	Fats
_________________________				
_________________________				
_________________________				
_________________________				

Snacks

	Calories	Carbs	Protein	Fats
_________________________				
_________________________				
_________________________				
_________________________				

Dinner

	Calories	Carbs	Protein	Fats
_________________________				
_________________________				
_________________________				
_________________________				

	Calories	Carbs	Protein	Fats
Totals				

Cups of Water Today

Date: _______________________

Breakfast

	Calories	Carbs	Protein	Fats
_______________	☐	☐	☐	☐
_______________	☐	☐	☐	☐
_______________	☐	☐	☐	☐
_______________	☐	☐	☐	☐

Lunch

	Calories	Carbs	Protein	Fats
_______________	☐	☐	☐	☐
_______________	☐	☐	☐	☐
_______________	☐	☐	☐	☐
_______________	☐	☐	☐	☐

Snacks

	Calories	Carbs	Protein	Fats
_______________	☐	☐	☐	☐
_______________	☐	☐	☐	☐
_______________	☐	☐	☐	☐
_______________	☐	☐	☐	☐

Dinner

	Calories	Carbs	Protein	Fats
_______________	☐	☐	☐	☐
_______________	☐	☐	☐	☐
_______________	☐	☐	☐	☐
_______________	☐	☐	☐	☐

	Calories	Carbs	Protein	Fats
Totals	☐	☐	☐	☐

Cups of Water Today

Date: _______________________

Breakfast

	Calories	Carbs	Protein	Fats
_______________________				
_______________________				
_______________________				
_______________________				

Lunch

	Calories	Carbs	Protein	Fats
_______________________				
_______________________				
_______________________				
_______________________				

Snacks

	Calories	Carbs	Protein	Fats
_______________________				
_______________________				
_______________________				
_______________________				

Dinner

	Calories	Carbs	Protein	Fats
_______________________				
_______________________				
_______________________				
_______________________				

	Calories	Carbs	Protein	Fats
Totals				

Cups of Water Today

Date: ______________________

Breakfast

	Calories	Carbs	Protein	Fats

____

____

____

____

Lunch

	Calories	Carbs	Protein	Fats

____

____

____

____

Snacks

	Calories	Carbs	Protein	Fats

____

____

____

____

Dinner

	Calories	Carbs	Protein	Fats

____

____

____

____

	Calories	Carbs	Protein	Fats
Totals				

Cups of Water Today

Date: _______________________

Breakfast

	Calories	Carbs	Protein	Fats
_______________________				
_______________________				
_______________________				
_______________________				

Lunch

	Calories	Carbs	Protein	Fats
_______________________				
_______________________				
_______________________				
_______________________				

Snacks

	Calories	Carbs	Protein	Fats
_______________________				
_______________________				
_______________________				
_______________________				

Dinner

	Calories	Carbs	Protein	Fats
_______________________				
_______________________				
_______________________				
_______________________				

	Calories	Carbs	Protein	Fats
Totals				

Cups of Water Today

Date: _______________________

Breakfast

	Calories	Carbs	Protein	Fats
____

____

____

____

Lunch

	Calories	Carbs	Protein	Fats
____

____

____

____

Snacks

	Calories	Carbs	Protein	Fats
____

____

____

____

Dinner

	Calories	Carbs	Protein	Fats
____

____

____

____

	Calories	Carbs	Protein	Fats
Totals				

Cups of Water Today

Date: _______________________

Breakfast

	Calories	Carbs	Protein	Fats
________________________				
________________________				
________________________				
________________________				

Lunch

	Calories	Carbs	Protein	Fats
________________________				
________________________				
________________________				
________________________				

Snacks

	Calories	Carbs	Protein	Fats
________________________				
________________________				
________________________				
________________________				

Dinner

	Calories	Carbs	Protein	Fats
________________________				
________________________				
________________________				
________________________				

	Calories	Carbs	Protein	Fats
Totals				

Cups of Water Today

Date: _______________________

Breakfast

	Calories	Carbs	Protein	Fats
_______________________				
_______________________				
_______________________				
_______________________				

Lunch

	Calories	Carbs	Protein	Fats
_______________________				
_______________________				
_______________________				
_______________________				

Snacks

	Calories	Carbs	Protein	Fats
_______________________				
_______________________				
_______________________				
_______________________				

Dinner

	Calories	Carbs	Protein	Fats
_______________________				
_______________________				
_______________________				
_______________________				

	Calories	Carbs	Protein	Fats
Totals				

Cups of Water Today

Date: _______________________

Breakfast

	Calories	Carbs	Protein	Fats
_____________________				
_____________________				
_____________________				
_____________________				

Lunch

	Calories	Carbs	Protein	Fats
_____________________				
_____________________				
_____________________				
_____________________				

Snacks

	Calories	Carbs	Protein	Fats
_____________________				
_____________________				
_____________________				
_____________________				

Dinner

	Calories	Carbs	Protein	Fats
_____________________				
_____________________				
_____________________				
_____________________				

	Calories	Carbs	Protein	Fats
Totals				

Cups of Water Today

Date: _______________________

Breakfast

	Calories	Carbs	Protein	Fats
____________________				
____________________				
____________________				
____________________				

Lunch

	Calories	Carbs	Protein	Fats
____________________				
____________________				
____________________				
____________________				

Snacks

	Calories	Carbs	Protein	Fats
____________________				
____________________				
____________________				
____________________				

Dinner

	Calories	Carbs	Protein	Fats
____________________				
____________________				
____________________				
____________________				

	Calories	Carbs	Protein	Fats
Totals				

Cups of Water Today

Date: _______________________

Breakfast

	Calories	Carbs	Protein	Fats
_________________________				
_________________________				
_________________________				
_________________________				

Lunch

	Calories	Carbs	Protein	Fats
_________________________				
_________________________				
_________________________				
_________________________				

Snacks

	Calories	Carbs	Protein	Fats
_________________________				
_________________________				
_________________________				
_________________________				

Dinner

	Calories	Carbs	Protein	Fats
_________________________				
_________________________				
_________________________				
_________________________				

	Calories	Carbs	Protein	Fats
Totals				

Cups of Water Today

Date: ___________________________

Breakfast

	Calories	Carbs	Protein	Fats
____________________				
____________________				
____________________				
____________________				

Lunch

	Calories	Carbs	Protein	Fats
____________________				
____________________				
____________________				
____________________				

Snacks

	Calories	Carbs	Protein	Fats
____________________				
____________________				
____________________				
____________________				

Dinner

	Calories	Carbs	Protein	Fats
____________________				
____________________				
____________________				
____________________				

	Calories	Carbs	Protein	Fats
Totals				

Cups of Water Today

Date: _______________________

Breakfast

	Calories	Carbs	Protein	Fats
_________________________				
_________________________				
_________________________				
_________________________				

Lunch

	Calories	Carbs	Protein	Fats
_________________________				
_________________________				
_________________________				
_________________________				

Snacks

	Calories	Carbs	Protein	Fats
_________________________				
_________________________				
_________________________				
_________________________				

Dinner

	Calories	Carbs	Protein	Fats
_________________________				
_________________________				
_________________________				
_________________________				

	Calories	Carbs	Protein	Fats
Totals				

Cups of Water Today

Date: ________________________

Breakfast

	Calories	Carbs	Protein	Fats
___________________________				
___________________________				
___________________________				
___________________________				

Lunch

	Calories	Carbs	Protein	Fats
___________________________				
___________________________				
___________________________				
___________________________				

Snacks

	Calories	Carbs	Protein	Fats
___________________________				
___________________________				
___________________________				
___________________________				

Dinner

	Calories	Carbs	Protein	Fats
___________________________				
___________________________				
___________________________				
___________________________				

	Calories	Carbs	Protein	Fats
Totals				

Cups of Water Today

Date: _______________________

Breakfast

	Calories	Carbs	Protein	Fats
________________________				
________________________				
________________________				
________________________				

Lunch

	Calories	Carbs	Protein	Fats
________________________				
________________________				
________________________				
________________________				

Snacks

	Calories	Carbs	Protein	Fats
________________________				
________________________				
________________________				
________________________				

Dinner

	Calories	Carbs	Protein	Fats
________________________				
________________________				
________________________				
________________________				

	Calories	Carbs	Protein	Fats
Totals				

Cups of Water Today

Date: ______________________

Breakfast

	Calories	Carbs	Protein	Fats
________________				
________________				
________________				
________________				

Lunch

	Calories	Carbs	Protein	Fats
________________				
________________				
________________				
________________				

Snacks

	Calories	Carbs	Protein	Fats
________________				
________________				
________________				
________________				

Dinner

	Calories	Carbs	Protein	Fats
________________				
________________				
________________				
________________				

	Calories	Carbs	Protein	Fats
Totals				

Cups of Water Today

Date: _______________________

Breakfast

	Calories	Carbs	Protein	Fats
_______________				
_______________				
_______________				
_______________				

Lunch

	Calories	Carbs	Protein	Fats
_______________				
_______________				
_______________				
_______________				

Snacks

	Calories	Carbs	Protein	Fats
_______________				
_______________				
_______________				
_______________				

Dinner

	Calories	Carbs	Protein	Fats
_______________				
_______________				
_______________				
_______________				

	Calories	Carbs	Protein	Fats
Totals				

Cups of Water Today

Date: ______________________

Breakfast

	Calories	Carbs	Protein	Fats
______________________				
______________________				
______________________				
______________________				

Lunch

	Calories	Carbs	Protein	Fats
______________________				
______________________				
______________________				
______________________				

Snacks

	Calories	Carbs	Protein	Fats
______________________				
______________________				
______________________				
______________________				

Dinner

	Calories	Carbs	Protein	Fats
______________________				
______________________				
______________________				
______________________				

	Calories	Carbs	Protein	Fats
Totals				

Cups of Water Today

Date: _______________________

Breakfast

	Calories	Carbs	Protein	Fats
__________________________	☐	☐	☐	☐
__________________________	☐	☐	☐	☐
__________________________	☐	☐	☐	☐
__________________________	☐	☐	☐	☐

Lunch

	Calories	Carbs	Protein	Fats
__________________________	☐	☐	☐	☐
__________________________	☐	☐	☐	☐
__________________________	☐	☐	☐	☐
__________________________	☐	☐	☐	☐

Snacks

	Calories	Carbs	Protein	Fats
__________________________	☐	☐	☐	☐
__________________________	☐	☐	☐	☐
__________________________	☐	☐	☐	☐
__________________________	☐	☐	☐	☐

Dinner

	Calories	Carbs	Protein	Fats
__________________________	☐	☐	☐	☐
__________________________	☐	☐	☐	☐
__________________________	☐	☐	☐	☐
__________________________	☐	☐	☐	☐

	Calories	Carbs	Protein	Fats
Totals	☐	☐	☐	☐

Cups of Water Today

Date: ______________________

Breakfast

	Calories	Carbs	Protein	Fats
______________________				
______________________				
______________________				
______________________				

Lunch

	Calories	Carbs	Protein	Fats
______________________				
______________________				
______________________				
______________________				

Snacks

	Calories	Carbs	Protein	Fats
______________________				
______________________				
______________________				
______________________				

Dinner

	Calories	Carbs	Protein	Fats
______________________				
______________________				
______________________				
______________________				

	Calories	Carbs	Protein	Fats
Totals				

Cups of Water Today

Date: _______________________

Breakfast

	Calories	Carbs	Protein	Fats
_____________________	☐	☐	☐	☐
_____________________	☐	☐	☐	☐
_____________________	☐	☐	☐	☐
_____________________	☐	☐	☐	☐

Lunch

	Calories	Carbs	Protein	Fats
_____________________	☐	☐	☐	☐
_____________________	☐	☐	☐	☐
_____________________	☐	☐	☐	☐
_____________________	☐	☐	☐	☐

Snacks

	Calories	Carbs	Protein	Fats
_____________________	☐	☐	☐	☐
_____________________	☐	☐	☐	☐
_____________________	☐	☐	☐	☐
_____________________	☐	☐	☐	☐

Dinner

	Calories	Carbs	Protein	Fats
_____________________	☐	☐	☐	☐
_____________________	☐	☐	☐	☐
_____________________	☐	☐	☐	☐
_____________________	☐	☐	☐	☐

	Calories	Carbs	Protein	Fats
Totals	☐	☐	☐	☐

Cups of Water Today

Date: ____________________________

Breakfast

	Calories	Carbs	Protein	Fats
______________________________				
______________________________				
______________________________				
______________________________				

Lunch

	Calories	Carbs	Protein	Fats
______________________________				
______________________________				
______________________________				
______________________________				

Snacks

	Calories	Carbs	Protein	Fats
______________________________				
______________________________				
______________________________				
______________________________				

Dinner

	Calories	Carbs	Protein	Fats
______________________________				
______________________________				
______________________________				
______________________________				

	Calories	Carbs	Protein	Fats
Totals				

Cups of Water Today

Date: ___________________________

Breakfast

	Calories	Carbs	Protein	Fats
_________________________				
_________________________				
_________________________				
_________________________				

Lunch

	Calories	Carbs	Protein	Fats
_________________________				
_________________________				
_________________________				
_________________________				

Snacks

	Calories	Carbs	Protein	Fats
_________________________				
_________________________				
_________________________				
_________________________				

Dinner

	Calories	Carbs	Protein	Fats
_________________________				
_________________________				
_________________________				
_________________________				

	Calories	Carbs	Protein	Fats
Totals				

Cups of Water Today

Date: ___________________________

Breakfast

	Calories	Carbs	Protein	Fats
__________________				
__________________				
__________________				
__________________				

Lunch

	Calories	Carbs	Protein	Fats
__________________				
__________________				
__________________				
__________________				

Snacks

	Calories	Carbs	Protein	Fats
__________________				
__________________				
__________________				
__________________				

Dinner

	Calories	Carbs	Protein	Fats
__________________				
__________________				
__________________				
__________________				

	Calories	Carbs	Protein	Fats
Totals				

Cups of Water Today

Date: ________________________

Breakfast

	Calories	Carbs	Protein	Fats
__________________________				
__________________________				
__________________________				
__________________________				

Lunch

	Calories	Carbs	Protein	Fats
__________________________				
__________________________				
__________________________				
__________________________				

Snacks

	Calories	Carbs	Protein	Fats
__________________________				
__________________________				
__________________________				
__________________________				

Dinner

	Calories	Carbs	Protein	Fats
__________________________				
__________________________				
__________________________				
__________________________				

	Calories	Carbs	Protein	Fats
Totals				

Cups of Water Today

Date: ______________________

Breakfast

	Calories	Carbs	Protein	Fats
___________________				
___________________				
___________________				
___________________				

Lunch

	Calories	Carbs	Protein	Fats
___________________				
___________________				
___________________				
___________________				

Snacks

	Calories	Carbs	Protein	Fats
___________________				
___________________				
___________________				
___________________				

Dinner

	Calories	Carbs	Protein	Fats
___________________				
___________________				
___________________				
___________________				

	Calories	Carbs	Protein	Fats
Totals				

Cups of Water Today

Date: _______________________

Breakfast

	Calories	Carbs	Protein	Fats
_______________________	☐	☐	☐	☐
_______________________	☐	☐	☐	☐
_______________________	☐	☐	☐	☐
_______________________	☐	☐	☐	☐

Lunch

	Calories	Carbs	Protein	Fats
_______________________	☐	☐	☐	☐
_______________________	☐	☐	☐	☐
_______________________	☐	☐	☐	☐
_______________________	☐	☐	☐	☐

Snacks

	Calories	Carbs	Protein	Fats
_______________________	☐	☐	☐	☐
_______________________	☐	☐	☐	☐
_______________________	☐	☐	☐	☐
_______________________	☐	☐	☐	☐

Dinner

	Calories	Carbs	Protein	Fats
_______________________	☐	☐	☐	☐
_______________________	☐	☐	☐	☐
_______________________	☐	☐	☐	☐
_______________________	☐	☐	☐	☐

	Calories	Carbs	Protein	Fats
Totals	☐	☐	☐	☐

Cups of Water Today

Date: _______________________

Breakfast

	Calories	Carbs	Protein	Fats
____________________				
____________________				
____________________				
____________________				

Lunch

	Calories	Carbs	Protein	Fats
____________________				
____________________				
____________________				
____________________				

Snacks

	Calories	Carbs	Protein	Fats
____________________				
____________________				
____________________				
____________________				

Dinner

	Calories	Carbs	Protein	Fats
____________________				
____________________				
____________________				
____________________				

	Calories	Carbs	Protein	Fats
Totals				

Cups of Water Today

Date: _______________________

Breakfast

	Calories	Carbs	Protein	Fats
_________________________				
_________________________				
_________________________				
_________________________				

Lunch

	Calories	Carbs	Protein	Fats
_________________________				
_________________________				
_________________________				
_________________________				

Snacks

	Calories	Carbs	Protein	Fats
_________________________				
_________________________				
_________________________				
_________________________				

Dinner

	Calories	Carbs	Protein	Fats
_________________________				
_________________________				
_________________________				
_________________________				

	Calories	Carbs	Protein	Fats
Totals				

Cups of Water Today

Date: ______________________

Breakfast

	Calories	Carbs	Protein	Fats
________________________				
________________________				
________________________				
________________________				

Lunch

	Calories	Carbs	Protein	Fats
________________________				
________________________				
________________________				
________________________				

Snacks

	Calories	Carbs	Protein	Fats
________________________				
________________________				
________________________				
________________________				

Dinner

	Calories	Carbs	Protein	Fats
________________________				
________________________				
________________________				
________________________				

	Calories	Carbs	Protein	Fats
Totals				

Cups of Water Today

Date: _______________________

Breakfast

	Calories	Carbs	Protein	Fats
_______________________				
_______________________				
_______________________				
_______________________				

Lunch

	Calories	Carbs	Protein	Fats
_______________________				
_______________________				
_______________________				
_______________________				

Snacks

	Calories	Carbs	Protein	Fats
_______________________				
_______________________				
_______________________				
_______________________				

Dinner

	Calories	Carbs	Protein	Fats
_______________________				
_______________________				
_______________________				
_______________________				

	Calories	Carbs	Protein	Fats
Totals				

Cups of Water Today

Date: ________________________

Breakfast

	Calories	Carbs	Protein	Fats
________________________				
________________________				
________________________				
________________________				

Lunch

	Calories	Carbs	Protein	Fats
________________________				
________________________				
________________________				
________________________				

Snacks

	Calories	Carbs	Protein	Fats
________________________				
________________________				
________________________				
________________________				

Dinner

	Calories	Carbs	Protein	Fats
________________________				
________________________				
________________________				
________________________				

	Calories	Carbs	Protein	Fats
Totals				

Cups of Water Today

Date: _______________________________

Breakfast

	Calories	Carbs	Protein	Fats
________________________________	☐	☐	☐	☐
________________________________	☐	☐	☐	☐
________________________________	☐	☐	☐	☐
________________________________	☐	☐	☐	☐

Lunch

	Calories	Carbs	Protein	Fats
________________________________	☐	☐	☐	☐
________________________________	☐	☐	☐	☐
________________________________	☐	☐	☐	☐
________________________________	☐	☐	☐	☐

Snacks

	Calories	Carbs	Protein	Fats
________________________________	☐	☐	☐	☐
________________________________	☐	☐	☐	☐
________________________________	☐	☐	☐	☐
________________________________	☐	☐	☐	☐

Dinner

	Calories	Carbs	Protein	Fats
________________________________	☐	☐	☐	☐
________________________________	☐	☐	☐	☐
________________________________	☐	☐	☐	☐
________________________________	☐	☐	☐	☐

	Calories	Carbs	Protein	Fats
Totals	☐	☐	☐	☐

Cups of Water Today

Date: ______________________

Breakfast

	Calories	Carbs	Protein	Fats
______________________				
______________________				
______________________				
______________________				

Lunch

	Calories	Carbs	Protein	Fats
______________________				
______________________				
______________________				
______________________				

Snacks

	Calories	Carbs	Protein	Fats
______________________				
______________________				
______________________				
______________________				

Dinner

	Calories	Carbs	Protein	Fats
______________________				
______________________				
______________________				
______________________				

	Calories	Carbs	Protein	Fats
Totals				

Cups of Water Today

Date: _______________________

Breakfast

	Calories	Carbs	Protein	Fats
_________________________				
_________________________				
_________________________				
_________________________				

Lunch

	Calories	Carbs	Protein	Fats
_________________________				
_________________________				
_________________________				
_________________________				

Snacks

	Calories	Carbs	Protein	Fats
_________________________				
_________________________				
_________________________				
_________________________				

Dinner

	Calories	Carbs	Protein	Fats
_________________________				
_________________________				
_________________________				
_________________________				

	Calories	Carbs	Protein	Fats
Totals				

Cups of Water Today

Date: ___________________________

Breakfast

	Calories	Carbs	Protein	Fats
___________________________				
___________________________				
___________________________				
___________________________				

Lunch

	Calories	Carbs	Protein	Fats
___________________________				
___________________________				
___________________________				
___________________________				

Snacks

	Calories	Carbs	Protein	Fats
___________________________				
___________________________				
___________________________				
___________________________				

Dinner

	Calories	Carbs	Protein	Fats
___________________________				
___________________________				
___________________________				
___________________________				

	Calories	Carbs	Protein	Fats
Totals				

Cups of Water Today

Date: _______________________

Breakfast

	Calories	Carbs	Protein	Fats
_________________________				
_________________________				
_________________________				
_________________________				

Lunch

	Calories	Carbs	Protein	Fats
_________________________				
_________________________				
_________________________				
_________________________				

Snacks

	Calories	Carbs	Protein	Fats
_________________________				
_________________________				
_________________________				
_________________________				

Dinner

	Calories	Carbs	Protein	Fats
_________________________				
_________________________				
_________________________				
_________________________				

	Calories	Carbs	Protein	Fats
Totals				

Cups of Water Today

Date: ___________________________

Breakfast

	Calories	Carbs	Protein	Fats
_______________________				
_______________________				
_______________________				
_______________________				

Lunch

	Calories	Carbs	Protein	Fats
_______________________				
_______________________				
_______________________				
_______________________				

Snacks

	Calories	Carbs	Protein	Fats
_______________________				
_______________________				
_______________________				
_______________________				

Dinner

	Calories	Carbs	Protein	Fats
_______________________				
_______________________				
_______________________				
_______________________				

	Calories	Carbs	Protein	Fats
Totals				

Cups of Water Today

Date: ______________________

Breakfast

	Calories	Carbs	Protein	Fats
_____________________				
_____________________				
_____________________				
_____________________				

Lunch

	Calories	Carbs	Protein	Fats
_____________________				
_____________________				
_____________________				
_____________________				

Snacks

	Calories	Carbs	Protein	Fats
_____________________				
_____________________				
_____________________				
_____________________				

Dinner

	Calories	Carbs	Protein	Fats
_____________________				
_____________________				
_____________________				
_____________________				

	Calories	Carbs	Protein	Fats
Totals				

Cups of Water Today

Date: ______________________

Breakfast

	Calories	Carbs	Protein	Fats
____________________	☐	☐	☐	☐
____________________	☐	☐	☐	☐
____________________	☐	☐	☐	☐
____________________	☐	☐	☐	☐

Lunch

	Calories	Carbs	Protein	Fats
____________________	☐	☐	☐	☐
____________________	☐	☐	☐	☐
____________________	☐	☐	☐	☐
____________________	☐	☐	☐	☐

Snacks

	Calories	Carbs	Protein	Fats
____________________	☐	☐	☐	☐
____________________	☐	☐	☐	☐
____________________	☐	☐	☐	☐
____________________	☐	☐	☐	☐

Dinner

	Calories	Carbs	Protein	Fats
____________________	☐	☐	☐	☐
____________________	☐	☐	☐	☐
____________________	☐	☐	☐	☐
____________________	☐	☐	☐	☐

	Calories	Carbs	Protein	Fats
Totals	☐	☐	☐	☐

Cups of Water Today

Date: _______________________

Breakfast

	Calories	Carbs	Protein	Fats
_________________________				
_________________________				
_________________________				
_________________________				

Lunch

	Calories	Carbs	Protein	Fats
_________________________				
_________________________				
_________________________				
_________________________				

Snacks

	Calories	Carbs	Protein	Fats
_________________________				
_________________________				
_________________________				
_________________________				

Dinner

	Calories	Carbs	Protein	Fats
_________________________				
_________________________				
_________________________				
_________________________				

	Calories	Carbs	Protein	Fats
Totals				

Cups of Water Today

Date: ___________________________

Breakfast

	Calories	Carbs	Protein	Fats
_______________________				
_______________________				
_______________________				
_______________________				

Lunch

	Calories	Carbs	Protein	Fats
_______________________				
_______________________				
_______________________				
_______________________				

Snacks

	Calories	Carbs	Protein	Fats
_______________________				
_______________________				
_______________________				
_______________________				

Dinner

	Calories	Carbs	Protein	Fats
_______________________				
_______________________				
_______________________				
_______________________				

	Calories	Carbs	Protein	Fats
Totals				

Cups of Water Today

Date: _______________________

Breakfast

	Calories	Carbs	Protein	Fats
_________________________				
_________________________				
_________________________				
_________________________				

Lunch

	Calories	Carbs	Protein	Fats
_________________________				
_________________________				
_________________________				
_________________________				

Snacks

	Calories	Carbs	Protein	Fats
_________________________				
_________________________				
_________________________				
_________________________				

Dinner

	Calories	Carbs	Protein	Fats
_________________________				
_________________________				
_________________________				
_________________________				

	Calories	Carbs	Protein	Fats
Totals				

Cups of Water Today

Date: _______________________

Breakfast

	Calories	Carbs	Protein	Fats
_____________________	☐	☐	☐	☐
_____________________	☐	☐	☐	☐
_____________________	☐	☐	☐	☐
_____________________	☐	☐	☐	☐

Lunch

	Calories	Carbs	Protein	Fats
_____________________	☐	☐	☐	☐
_____________________	☐	☐	☐	☐
_____________________	☐	☐	☐	☐
_____________________	☐	☐	☐	☐

Snacks

	Calories	Carbs	Protein	Fats
_____________________	☐	☐	☐	☐
_____________________	☐	☐	☐	☐
_____________________	☐	☐	☐	☐
_____________________	☐	☐	☐	☐

Dinner

	Calories	Carbs	Protein	Fats
_____________________	☐	☐	☐	☐
_____________________	☐	☐	☐	☐
_____________________	☐	☐	☐	☐
_____________________	☐	☐	☐	☐

	Calories	Carbs	Protein	Fats
Totals	☐	☐	☐	☐

Cups of Water Today

Date: _______________________

Breakfast

	Calories	Carbs	Protein	Fats
_________________				
_________________				
_________________				
_________________				

Lunch

	Calories	Carbs	Protein	Fats
_________________				
_________________				
_________________				
_________________				

Snacks

	Calories	Carbs	Protein	Fats
_________________				
_________________				
_________________				
_________________				

Dinner

	Calories	Carbs	Protein	Fats
_________________				
_________________				
_________________				
_________________				

	Calories	Carbs	Protein	Fats
Totals				

Cups of Water Today

Date: _______________________

Breakfast

	Calories	Carbs	Protein	Fats
_________________________				
_________________________				
_________________________				
_________________________				

Lunch

	Calories	Carbs	Protein	Fats
_________________________				
_________________________				
_________________________				
_________________________				

Snacks

	Calories	Carbs	Protein	Fats
_________________________				
_________________________				
_________________________				
_________________________				

Dinner

	Calories	Carbs	Protein	Fats
_________________________				
_________________________				
_________________________				
_________________________				

	Calories	Carbs	Protein	Fats
Totals				

Cups of Water Today

Date: _______________________

Breakfast

	Calories	Carbs	Protein	Fats
_______________________				
_______________________				
_______________________				
_______________________				

Lunch

	Calories	Carbs	Protein	Fats
_______________________				
_______________________				
_______________________				
_______________________				

Snacks

	Calories	Carbs	Protein	Fats
_______________________				
_______________________				
_______________________				
_______________________				

Dinner

	Calories	Carbs	Protein	Fats
_______________________				
_______________________				
_______________________				
_______________________				

	Calories	Carbs	Protein	Fats
Totals				

Cups of Water Today

Date: ___________________________

Breakfast

	Calories	Carbs	Protein	Fats
________________________				
________________________				
________________________				
________________________				

Lunch

	Calories	Carbs	Protein	Fats
________________________				
________________________				
________________________				
________________________				

Snacks

	Calories	Carbs	Protein	Fats
________________________				
________________________				
________________________				
________________________				

Dinner

	Calories	Carbs	Protein	Fats
________________________				
________________________				
________________________				
________________________				

	Calories	Carbs	Protein	Fats
Totals				

Cups of Water Today

Date: _______________________

Breakfast

	Calories	Carbs	Protein	Fats
_________________________				
_________________________				
_________________________				
_________________________				

Lunch

	Calories	Carbs	Protein	Fats
_________________________				
_________________________				
_________________________				
_________________________				

Snacks

	Calories	Carbs	Protein	Fats
_________________________				
_________________________				
_________________________				
_________________________				

Dinner

	Calories	Carbs	Protein	Fats
_________________________				
_________________________				
_________________________				
_________________________				

	Calories	Carbs	Protein	Fats
Totals				

Cups of Water Today

Date: ___________________________

Breakfast

	Calories	Carbs	Protein	Fats
____________________				
____________________				
____________________				
____________________				

Lunch

	Calories	Carbs	Protein	Fats
____________________				
____________________				
____________________				
____________________				

Snacks

	Calories	Carbs	Protein	Fats
____________________				
____________________				
____________________				
____________________				

Dinner

	Calories	Carbs	Protein	Fats
____________________				
____________________				
____________________				
____________________				

	Calories	Carbs	Protein	Fats
Totals				

Cups of Water Today

Date: ______________________

Breakfast

	Calories	Carbs	Protein	Fats
__________________				
__________________				
__________________				
__________________				

Lunch

	Calories	Carbs	Protein	Fats
__________________				
__________________				
__________________				
__________________				

Snacks

	Calories	Carbs	Protein	Fats
__________________				
__________________				
__________________				
__________________				

Dinner

	Calories	Carbs	Protein	Fats
__________________				
__________________				
__________________				
__________________				

	Calories	Carbs	Protein	Fats
Totals				

Cups of Water Today

Date: _______________________

Breakfast

	Calories	Carbs	Protein	Fats
_____________________				
_____________________				
_____________________				
_____________________				

Lunch

	Calories	Carbs	Protein	Fats
_____________________				
_____________________				
_____________________				
_____________________				

Snacks

	Calories	Carbs	Protein	Fats
_____________________				
_____________________				
_____________________				
_____________________				

Dinner

	Calories	Carbs	Protein	Fats
_____________________				
_____________________				
_____________________				
_____________________				

	Calories	Carbs	Protein	Fats
Totals				

Cups of Water Today

Date: _______________________

Breakfast

	Calories	Carbs	Protein	Fats
_______________________				
_______________________				
_______________________				
_______________________				

Lunch

	Calories	Carbs	Protein	Fats
_______________________				
_______________________				
_______________________				
_______________________				

Snacks

	Calories	Carbs	Protein	Fats
_______________________				
_______________________				
_______________________				
_______________________				

Dinner

	Calories	Carbs	Protein	Fats
_______________________				
_______________________				
_______________________				
_______________________				

	Calories	Carbs	Protein	Fats
Totals				

Cups of Water Today

Date: _______________________

Breakfast

	Calories	Carbs	Protein	Fats
___________________				
___________________				
___________________				
___________________				

Lunch

	Calories	Carbs	Protein	Fats
___________________				
___________________				
___________________				
___________________				

Snacks

	Calories	Carbs	Protein	Fats
___________________				
___________________				
___________________				
___________________				

Dinner

	Calories	Carbs	Protein	Fats
___________________				
___________________				
___________________				
___________________				

	Calories	Carbs	Protein	Fats
Totals				

Cups of Water Today

Date: _______________________

Breakfast

	Calories	Carbs	Protein	Fats
_____________________				
_____________________				
_____________________				
_____________________				

Lunch

	Calories	Carbs	Protein	Fats
_____________________				
_____________________				
_____________________				
_____________________				

Snacks

	Calories	Carbs	Protein	Fats
_____________________				
_____________________				
_____________________				
_____________________				

Dinner

	Calories	Carbs	Protein	Fats
_____________________				
_____________________				
_____________________				
_____________________				

	Calories	Carbs	Protein	Fats
Totals				

Cups of Water Today

Date: _______________________

Breakfast

	Calories	Carbs	Protein	Fats
_____________				
_____________				
_____________				
_____________				

Lunch

	Calories	Carbs	Protein	Fats
_____________				
_____________				
_____________				
_____________				

Snacks

	Calories	Carbs	Protein	Fats
_____________				
_____________				
_____________				
_____________				

Dinner

	Calories	Carbs	Protein	Fats
_____________				
_____________				
_____________				
_____________				

	Calories	Carbs	Protein	Fats
Totals				

Cups of Water Today

Date: _______________________

Breakfast

	Calories	Carbs	Protein	Fats
____________________				
____________________				
____________________				
____________________				

Lunch

	Calories	Carbs	Protein	Fats
____________________				
____________________				
____________________				
____________________				

Snacks

	Calories	Carbs	Protein	Fats
____________________				
____________________				
____________________				
____________________				

Dinner

	Calories	Carbs	Protein	Fats
____________________				
____________________				
____________________				
____________________				

	Calories	Carbs	Protein	Fats
Totals				

Cups of Water Today

Date: ______________________

Breakfast

	Calories	Carbs	Protein	Fats
_______________________				
_______________________				
_______________________				
_______________________				

Lunch

	Calories	Carbs	Protein	Fats
_______________________				
_______________________				
_______________________				
_______________________				

Snacks

	Calories	Carbs	Protein	Fats
_______________________				
_______________________				
_______________________				
_______________________				

Dinner

	Calories	Carbs	Protein	Fats
_______________________				
_______________________				
_______________________				
_______________________				

	Calories	Carbs	Protein	Fats
Totals				

Cups of Water Today

Date: _______________________

Breakfast

	Calories	Carbs	Protein	Fats
_______________________				
_______________________				
_______________________				
_______________________				

Lunch

	Calories	Carbs	Protein	Fats
_______________________				
_______________________				
_______________________				
_______________________				

Snacks

	Calories	Carbs	Protein	Fats
_______________________				
_______________________				
_______________________				
_______________________				

Dinner

	Calories	Carbs	Protein	Fats
_______________________				
_______________________				
_______________________				
_______________________				

	Calories	Carbs	Protein	Fats
Totals				

Cups of Water Today

Date: ___________________________

Breakfast

	Calories	Carbs	Protein	Fats
____________________				
____________________				
____________________				
____________________				

Lunch

	Calories	Carbs	Protein	Fats
____________________				
____________________				
____________________				
____________________				

Snacks

	Calories	Carbs	Protein	Fats
____________________				
____________________				
____________________				
____________________				

Dinner

	Calories	Carbs	Protein	Fats
____________________				
____________________				
____________________				
____________________				

	Calories	Carbs	Protein	Fats
Totals				

Cups of Water Today

Date: _______________________

Breakfast

	Calories	Carbs	Protein	Fats
____________________				
____________________				
____________________				
____________________				

Lunch

	Calories	Carbs	Protein	Fats
____________________				
____________________				
____________________				
____________________				

Snacks

	Calories	Carbs	Protein	Fats
____________________				
____________________				
____________________				
____________________				

Dinner

	Calories	Carbs	Protein	Fats
____________________				
____________________				
____________________				
____________________				

	Calories	Carbs	Protein	Fats
Totals				

Cups of Water Today

Date: ________________________

Breakfast

	Calories	Carbs	Protein	Fats

Lunch

	Calories	Carbs	Protein	Fats

Snacks

	Calories	Carbs	Protein	Fats

Dinner

	Calories	Carbs	Protein	Fats

	Calories	Carbs	Protein	Fats
Totals				

Cups of Water Today

Date: _______________________

Breakfast

	Calories	Carbs	Protein	Fats
_________________________				
_________________________				
_________________________				
_________________________				

Lunch

	Calories	Carbs	Protein	Fats
_________________________				
_________________________				
_________________________				
_________________________				

Snacks

	Calories	Carbs	Protein	Fats
_________________________				
_________________________				
_________________________				
_________________________				

Dinner

	Calories	Carbs	Protein	Fats
_________________________				
_________________________				
_________________________				
_________________________				

	Calories	Carbs	Protein	Fats
Totals				

Cups of Water Today

Date: ______________________

Breakfast

	Calories	Carbs	Protein	Fats
______________________				
______________________				
______________________				
______________________				

Lunch

	Calories	Carbs	Protein	Fats
______________________				
______________________				
______________________				
______________________				

Snacks

	Calories	Carbs	Protein	Fats
______________________				
______________________				
______________________				
______________________				

Dinner

	Calories	Carbs	Protein	Fats
______________________				
______________________				
______________________				
______________________				

	Calories	Carbs	Protein	Fats
Totals				

Cups of Water Today

Date: _______________________

Breakfast

	Calories	Carbs	Protein	Fats
_________________________				
_________________________				
_________________________				
_________________________				

Lunch

	Calories	Carbs	Protein	Fats
_________________________				
_________________________				
_________________________				
_________________________				

Snacks

	Calories	Carbs	Protein	Fats
_________________________				
_________________________				
_________________________				
_________________________				

Dinner

	Calories	Carbs	Protein	Fats
_________________________				
_________________________				
_________________________				
_________________________				

	Calories	Carbs	Protein	Fats
Totals				

Cups of Water Today

Date: ______________________________

Breakfast

	Calories	Carbs	Protein	Fats
______________________________				
______________________________				
______________________________				
______________________________				

Lunch

	Calories	Carbs	Protein	Fats
______________________________				
______________________________				
______________________________				
______________________________				

Snacks

	Calories	Carbs	Protein	Fats
______________________________				
______________________________				
______________________________				
______________________________				

Dinner

	Calories	Carbs	Protein	Fats
______________________________				
______________________________				
______________________________				
______________________________				

	Calories	Carbs	Protein	Fats
Totals				

Cups of Water Today

Date: _______________________

Breakfast

	Calories	Carbs	Protein	Fats
_________________________				
_________________________				
_________________________				
_________________________				

Lunch

	Calories	Carbs	Protein	Fats
_________________________				
_________________________				
_________________________				
_________________________				

Snacks

	Calories	Carbs	Protein	Fats
_________________________				
_________________________				
_________________________				
_________________________				

Dinner

	Calories	Carbs	Protein	Fats
_________________________				
_________________________				
_________________________				
_________________________				

	Calories	Carbs	Protein	Fats
Totals				

Cups of Water Today

Date: ___________________________

Breakfast

	Calories	Carbs	Protein	Fats
___________________________	☐	☐	☐	☐
___________________________	☐	☐	☐	☐
___________________________	☐	☐	☐	☐
___________________________	☐	☐	☐	☐

Lunch

	Calories	Carbs	Protein	Fats
___________________________	☐	☐	☐	☐
___________________________	☐	☐	☐	☐
___________________________	☐	☐	☐	☐
___________________________	☐	☐	☐	☐

Snacks

	Calories	Carbs	Protein	Fats
___________________________	☐	☐	☐	☐
___________________________	☐	☐	☐	☐
___________________________	☐	☐	☐	☐
___________________________	☐	☐	☐	☐

Dinner

	Calories	Carbs	Protein	Fats
___________________________	☐	☐	☐	☐
___________________________	☐	☐	☐	☐
___________________________	☐	☐	☐	☐
___________________________	☐	☐	☐	☐

	Calories	Carbs	Protein	Fats
Totals	☐	☐	☐	☐

Cups of Water Today

Date: _______________________

Breakfast

	Calories	Carbs	Protein	Fats
_______________________				
_______________________				
_______________________				
_______________________				

Lunch

	Calories	Carbs	Protein	Fats
_______________________				
_______________________				
_______________________				
_______________________				

Snacks

	Calories	Carbs	Protein	Fats
_______________________				
_______________________				
_______________________				
_______________________				

Dinner

	Calories	Carbs	Protein	Fats
_______________________				
_______________________				
_______________________				
_______________________				

	Calories	Carbs	Protein	Fats
Totals				

Cups of Water Today

Date: _______________________

Breakfast

	Calories	Carbs	Protein	Fats
________________________				
________________________				
________________________				
________________________				

Lunch

	Calories	Carbs	Protein	Fats
________________________				
________________________				
________________________				
________________________				

Snacks

	Calories	Carbs	Protein	Fats
________________________				
________________________				
________________________				
________________________				

Dinner

	Calories	Carbs	Protein	Fats
________________________				
________________________				
________________________				
________________________				

	Calories	Carbs	Protein	Fats
Totals				

Cups of Water Today

Date: _______________________

Breakfast

	Calories	Carbs	Protein	Fats
_________________________				
_________________________				
_________________________				
_________________________				

Lunch

	Calories	Carbs	Protein	Fats
_________________________				
_________________________				
_________________________				
_________________________				

Snacks

	Calories	Carbs	Protein	Fats
_________________________				
_________________________				
_________________________				
_________________________				

Dinner

	Calories	Carbs	Protein	Fats
_________________________				
_________________________				
_________________________				
_________________________				

	Calories	Carbs	Protein	Fats
Totals				

Cups of Water Today

Date: _______________________

Breakfast

	Calories	Carbs	Protein	Fats
__________________________				
__________________________				
__________________________				
__________________________				

Lunch

	Calories	Carbs	Protein	Fats
__________________________				
__________________________				
__________________________				
__________________________				

Snacks

	Calories	Carbs	Protein	Fats
__________________________				
__________________________				
__________________________				
__________________________				

Dinner

	Calories	Carbs	Protein	Fats
__________________________				
__________________________				
__________________________				
__________________________				

	Calories	Carbs	Protein	Fats
Totals				

Cups of Water Today

Date: ___________________________

Breakfast

	Calories	Carbs	Protein	Fats
____________________				
____________________				
____________________				
____________________				

Lunch

	Calories	Carbs	Protein	Fats
____________________				
____________________				
____________________				
____________________				

Snacks

	Calories	Carbs	Protein	Fats
____________________				
____________________				
____________________				
____________________				

Dinner

	Calories	Carbs	Protein	Fats
____________________				
____________________				
____________________				
____________________				

	Calories	Carbs	Protein	Fats
Totals				

Cups of Water Today

Date: ______________________

Breakfast

	Calories	Carbs	Protein	Fats
______________________				
______________________				
______________________				
______________________				

Lunch

	Calories	Carbs	Protein	Fats
______________________				
______________________				
______________________				
______________________				

Snacks

	Calories	Carbs	Protein	Fats
______________________				
______________________				
______________________				
______________________				

Dinner

	Calories	Carbs	Protein	Fats
______________________				
______________________				
______________________				
______________________				

	Calories	Carbs	Protein	Fats
Totals				

Cups of Water Today

Date: ______________________

Breakfast

	Calories	Carbs	Protein	Fats
__________________				
__________________				
__________________				
__________________				

Lunch

	Calories	Carbs	Protein	Fats
__________________				
__________________				
__________________				
__________________				

Snacks

	Calories	Carbs	Protein	Fats
__________________				
__________________				
__________________				
__________________				

Dinner

	Calories	Carbs	Protein	Fats
__________________				
__________________				
__________________				
__________________				

	Calories	Carbs	Protein	Fats
Totals				

Cups of Water Today

Date: ______________________

Breakfast

	Calories	Carbs	Protein	Fats
______________________				
______________________				
______________________				
______________________				

Lunch

	Calories	Carbs	Protein	Fats
______________________				
______________________				
______________________				
______________________				

Snacks

	Calories	Carbs	Protein	Fats
______________________				
______________________				
______________________				
______________________				

Dinner

	Calories	Carbs	Protein	Fats
______________________				
______________________				
______________________				
______________________				

	Calories	Carbs	Protein	Fats
Totals				

Cups of Water Today

Date: _______________________

Breakfast

	Calories	Carbs	Protein	Fats
_________________________				
_________________________				
_________________________				
_________________________				

Lunch

	Calories	Carbs	Protein	Fats
_________________________				
_________________________				
_________________________				
_________________________				

Snacks

	Calories	Carbs	Protein	Fats
_________________________				
_________________________				
_________________________				
_________________________				

Dinner

	Calories	Carbs	Protein	Fats
_________________________				
_________________________				
_________________________				
_________________________				

	Calories	Carbs	Protein	Fats
Totals				

Cups of Water Today

Date: ______________________________

Breakfast

	Calories	Carbs	Protein	Fats
____________________				
____________________				
____________________				
____________________				

Lunch

	Calories	Carbs	Protein	Fats
____________________				
____________________				
____________________				
____________________				

Snacks

	Calories	Carbs	Protein	Fats
____________________				
____________________				
____________________				
____________________				

Dinner

	Calories	Carbs	Protein	Fats
____________________				
____________________				
____________________				
____________________				

	Calories	Carbs	Protein	Fats
Totals				

Cups of Water Today

Date: ________________________

Breakfast

	Calories	Carbs	Protein	Fats
________________________	☐	☐	☐	☐
________________________	☐	☐	☐	☐
________________________	☐	☐	☐	☐
________________________	☐	☐	☐	☐

Lunch

	Calories	Carbs	Protein	Fats
________________________	☐	☐	☐	☐
________________________	☐	☐	☐	☐
________________________	☐	☐	☐	☐
________________________	☐	☐	☐	☐

Snacks

	Calories	Carbs	Protein	Fats
________________________	☐	☐	☐	☐
________________________	☐	☐	☐	☐
________________________	☐	☐	☐	☐
________________________	☐	☐	☐	☐

Dinner

	Calories	Carbs	Protein	Fats
________________________	☐	☐	☐	☐
________________________	☐	☐	☐	☐
________________________	☐	☐	☐	☐
________________________	☐	☐	☐	☐

	Calories	Carbs	Protein	Fats
Totals	☐	☐	☐	☐

Cups of Water Today

www.ingramcontent.com/pod-product-compliance
Lightning Source LLC
Chambersburg PA
CBHW031300250726

48655CB00005B/2289